Anti Inflammatory Diet

A Practical Guide to Fight Inflammation With Healthy Diet Action Plans

Stephany J. Greene

Table of Contents

Introduction

Chronic inflammation is epidemic in Western culture. If you are reading this book, it's likely because you are one of the 1 in 5 adults in the United States who suffer from the effects of chronic inflammation, and from chronic inflammatory diseases like diabetes and arthritis.

Inflammation is a natural bodily response, putting your body in overdrive to fight off infection and aid healing. But when inflammation goes on too long it can trigger or contribute to a number of other diseases, such as heart disease, diabetes, cancer and Alzheimer's. The increase in the prevalence to these diseases parallels the increase in inflammation in the general population.

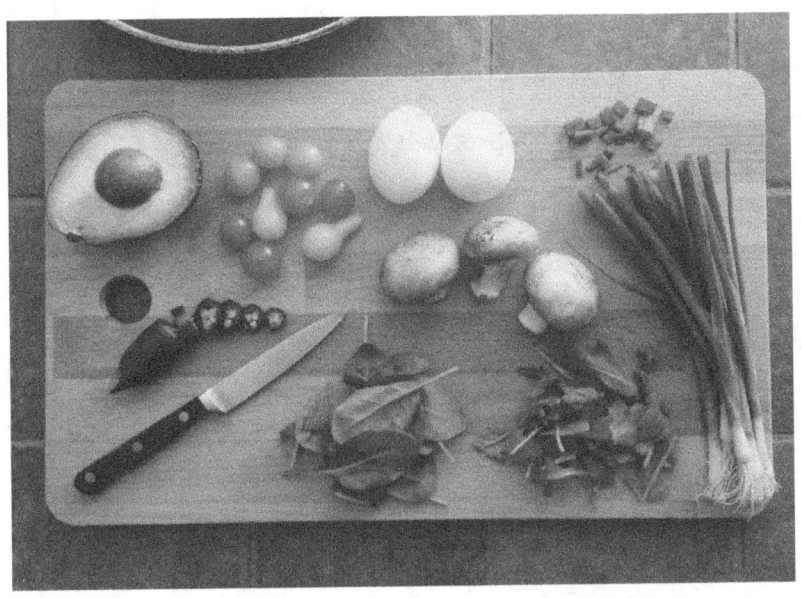

But here's the good news: *The choices you make in your life can significantly decrease inflammation in your body.* Medications for inflammation generally have a downside; but changes in your lifestyle and diet – changes you can make on your own, with the help of this book – can make a big difference in your life, with no corresponding challenges to your body or your well-being.

Because the choices we've made are a big factor in inflammation being such an issue today. Increased consumption of sugar and refined carbohydrates; a decrease in physical activity; increase in levels of obesity – all these choices have a huge impact on your body's inability to prevent chronic inflammation.

If you're experiencing constant pain and stiffness, problems regulating blood sugar, digestive discomfort, constant fatigue, or skin rashes associated with chronic inflammation, the information in this book could change your life. What's more – it could lead to a longer life, and bring you improvement that *makes life worth living*. Because struggling day after day with the issues inflammation brings into your life – that's no way to live.

There's a better life waiting for you, and it isn't that hard to achieve. I hope you'll use the guidelines in this book to make a difference in your health, and in the joy you find in life.

Inflammation – A Healthy Response Gone Bad

Having a basic knowledge on the topic of inflammation is the first step to solving the problems relating to it. Therefore, this chapter will investigate exactly what inflammation is, and what might cause this in your body. Although the causes are a little bit technical, I'll try my best for you to give you a good and understandable oversight.

Surprise: Inflammation is a Key to Good Health

Inflammation – you see the word everywhere, from articles on the pain and health challenges inflammation poses, to medications designed to address it. From the way we talk about inflammation, you wouldn't think it actually plays a much-needed role in staying healthy; but in fact, it does, at least until it gets out of control.

When your body is working as it should, inflammation is a useful and necessary response by your body's immune system. Acute inflammation – meaning, inflammation that comes and goes in response to injury - promotes healing. For example, when you cut yourself while cooking, the cut probably closes up with a scab, if it isn't too deep. In the next day or so, you may notice a little swelling, redness and heat – that's the presence of inflammation, fighting off viruses and infection. If all goes as it should, the swelling and redness disappear in a few days, the cut heals fully, and your finger is as good as new.

Acute inflammation's role in exercise even makes you healthier. The muscle soreness you feel after exercising is usually the result of small tears in the muscle that inflammation heals. The resulting healed muscle tissue is stronger than it was before, because of the inflammatory response.

When Things Go Wrong

Inflammation works well for us when it kicks in when needed – and stops when it's no longer needed, when healing is complete. *But when you continue to re-injure yourself, inflammation is constant,* and becomes "chronic".

It doesn't just happen if you continue to cut your finger again and again. Injuries that make the inflammatory response continue include severe lack of sleep; anxiety; and an inadequate amount of Omega-3 fats, and an excess of Omega-6 fats.

Another primary source of chronic inflammation is a constantly irritated gut lining that becomes inflammatory every time you eat. A little scary! Because even the strictest diet recognizes that you'll need to eat eventually. And if you have chronic gut irritation, that "eventually" turns into an inflammatory episode.

What it looks like in action? Check out an acute inflammation response of the body in the image below. Basically, it's your body's white blood cell's attacking what it sees as harmful intruders (which are the larger, weirdly shaped clusters in the middle and on the left side of the image).

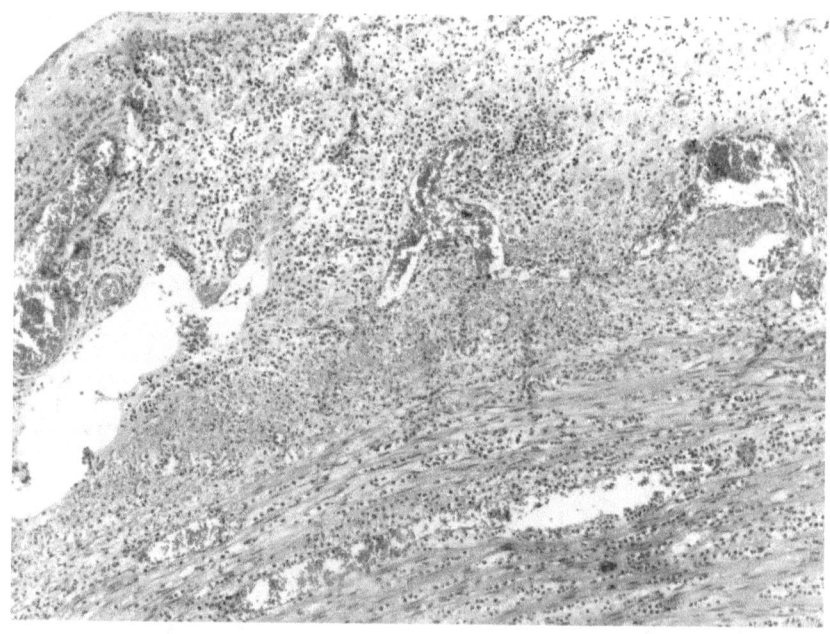

Tracking an Inflammatory Response

To understand chronic inflammation, it's following what an inflammatory response is like can really help.

At its root, inflammation is simply a way for our bodies to protect us from harmful *antigens*. The body's response to these alien substances consists of a series of actions, which together is what you experience as inflammation.

Step by step, these are the actions your body takes:

1. Your body is designed to protect you from *antigens*. Antigens are substances found on the surface of cells, bacteria and viruses. Your own cells have antigens as well. Your immune system has learned to recognize your own cellular antigens, and not attack – unless you have chronic inflammation.
2. Your body's first line of defense against antigens includes your skin, mucous membranes, coughing, enzymes in tears and oils, and stomach acid.
3. If an antigen gets past your body's line of defense, your immune system attacks and destroys it, with Lymphoctyes:
   - Lymphocyte B produces antibodies to attack antigens in your body;
   - Lymphocyte T attacks antigens directly.
4. The body increases the blood flow to the site of the antigens, which causes swelling. The swelling helps

isolate the antigen and keep it from spreading towards the rest of the body.

Chronic inflammation is an abnormal response to antigens. With chronic inflammation, once the antigen gets past the body's first line of defense, the body sends a signal to the immune system to attack antigens – but once the invading antigens are destroyed, the antibodies continue to attack the body itself. In some cases of chronic inflammation, the immune system creates antibodies even in the absence of an attack by antigens, and attacks internal organs and tissues.

Such attacks can be on specific organs, such as the thyroid (Hashimoto's thyroiditis and Graves' disease) or the pancreas, as with insulin-dependent diabetes mellitus, or IDDM. Systemic attacks from autoimmune conditions such as systemic lupus and primary Sjögren's syndrome, can affect a number of organs.

Causes of Chronic Inflammation

What are some of the possible causes chronic inflammation? Well, there's no real simple answer, as there are a combination of issues that might have caused it for you. And on top of that, a lot of possible causes are quite common with most people. You do not need to have all the causes in order to experience an inflammatory nuisance in your body. Let's take a look at them one by one.

Diet

Just as your skin works to keep foreign substances out – your mouth lets foreign or challenging substances in. Food allergies and intolerances cause an increase in inflammation (common ones are to gluten and casein).

Your body perceives the food as a foreign substance attacking your body, and your immune system attacks in return, resulting in inflammation. There are a number of approaches to addressing diet and inflammation in the last few chapters of this book.

Challenges to digestive system

When you eat more than your digestive system can handle, the digestive system goes into overdrive and results in inflammation. Red meat and sugar also challenge the digestive system, and can result in inflammation. Especially the consumption of such foods over long periods of time will result in health issues, when one is vulnerable to their effects.

Obesity

As white blood cells respond to swelling, healthy cells stop responding appropriately to insulin, resulting in diabetes and other issues. The diet suggestions in this book will support you in achieving your optimum weight.

Chronic stress

In response to stress, the brain takes actions that result in inflammation. Reducing stress is a whole topic for a book in itself, as most of the stress causes are different depending on your own life's situation. Some might experience stress in their home environment, because of their health situation, or because of excessively working.

In general, trying to reduce stress by breaking your regular schedule and living environment is a great way to reduce your stress levels.

Chemicals and pollution

The immune system is sensitive to changes and responds to chemicals and pollution, causing inflammation. Check if your environment could emit such substances into your own body, through the water, air or other means.

Chronic lack of sleep

Studies show insomniacs produce more cytokines, and cytokines increase inflammation. Sleeping more is also great to reduce stress, which is one of the other possible causes of inflammation.

Hormone imbalances

As hormonal activity fluctuates, inflammation results, causing menopausal women and others experiencing swings in hormonal activity to gain weight. Much attention is being given to the role chemicals and pollutants play in skewing hormone production, and thus resulting in inflammation.

Notice that in the list above, *all seven* causes are caused by or influenced by lifestyle choices. You needn't turn to medications – with dangerous side effects - to address inflammation. Diet and other lifestyle choices almost certainly had a major impact on your development of inflammation. Changing your diet and other lifestyle choices can have an enormous impact on healing your inflammation.

How Do You Know if You Have Chronic Inflammation?

In her mid-forties, Susan began to feel less vibrant. The change came on her so slowly that it was months before she began to recognize that something had changed. One morning, getting ready to go to work, she realized she just wanted to go back to bed; then she realized she had felt that way more mornings than not, for months. She began to have rashes, for no apparent reason. She began to have trouble completing her sentences, trouble remembering the word she was looking for. Often, she felt she was just moving through her life as through a soupy fog.

She began to seek medical help. The first doctor told her she was fine, just anemic. Another physician told her there was nothing really wrong, she just needed a Vitamin D supplement. The "just" diagnoses continued, doctor to doctor – while Susan felt worse and worse all the time. It was six years – *six years* –

before a physician diagnosed her with Hashimoto's Thyroiditis, an autoimmune disorder.

But that wasn't the end of Susan's struggle. The physician prescribed medication, which Susan took. She got worse instead of better, with joint pain, itching, and frequent bouts of dizziness. She began to feel that physicians and even friends and family doubted there was anything really wrong with her – that she was imagining her symptoms.

Like a lot of people with autoimmune, Susan never found a single physician, or a single treatment, that worked. And she never found a medication that really helped.

Instead, over the course of two years, she changed her food and lifestyle choices in a number of ways. She identified her food intolerances (gluten, corn and eggs) and – overwhelming as it seemed – began to eliminate them from her diet, for good. She increased foods high in fiber and antioxidants (such as eating blueberries). She ate probiotic foods and supplements. And she looked at the causes of stress in her life – like her job, and her mother – and, though it wasn't easy, she found another job that paid less but also stressed her out less. And she began, for the first time in her life, to draw boundaries with her mother.

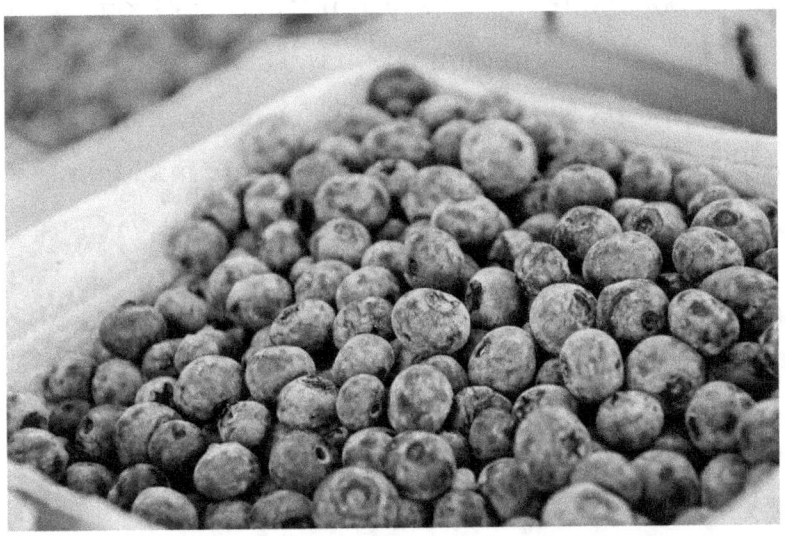

And she got better. Slowly at first. Then one day, she realized how much better she felt than she had a year ago. She continues to improve. There are flare-ups in which the aches and the brain fog return, mostly during allergy season, when her immune system is in overdrive. But she's better, and she recognizes it. And that gives her the will to keep to her anti-inflammatory protocol, and continue to look for new solutions.

Symptoms of Chronic Inflammation

How about you? If you're reading this book, you probably suspect inflammation is a challenge in your life. How do you know for sure? See if the following symptoms or possible indications of inflammation sound familiar.

- Allergies and asthma – have you struggled with allergies or had issues with asthma since you were a child? Allergy and asthma are both closely connected to inflammation.
- Ongoing aches and pains – if aches in muscles and joints are a regular element of your life, your body is almost certainly inflamed. The cytokines your immune cells or fat cells are producing make you feel sore and ache-y.
- Brain fog – do you feel you've been losing your ability to think clearly – to find the word you're looking for, to multi task as effectively as you used to?

- Overweight – if you're overweight, your fat cells are producing more inflammation-causing chemicals.

- Fatigue – one man with autoimmune said he began to realize he climbed two flights of stairs when he got to work – and he was done for the day. He just felt he might as well go home and go back to bed. If you're feeling more fatigued, much more often, inflammation could have a role in your struggle. If your immune system is producing too many inflammatory chemicals and antibodies, you may feel like you do when you are fighting off the flu – because as far as your immune system is concerned, you are.

- Skin problems – rashes, redness and itching are signs of inflammation.

- Infections – if you have chronic infections like hepatitis, herpes or *Epstein barr* virus, your body is in immune overdrive all the time – and that means inflammation.

- Allergies – if you suffer with allergies, you have the classic symptoms of inflammation: redness, swelling and itching. Allergies are experienced in response to substances that are *not* toxic (like pollen and certain foods), but that your body *perceives* as toxic. Exposing your body to them results in an immune response, and inflammation.

- Chronic digestive problems – if you have irritable bowel syndrome, ulcers, or frequently experience bloating, gas or diarrhea, it's a sign your gut is out of balance, and that almost always means there's inflammation.
- Trouble sleeping – chemicals and substances produced as a result of inflammation are also associated with sleep disorders, and a UCLA study links sleep disorders with inflammatory markers.
- You've been diagnosed with an autoimmune disease – any autoimmune disease results in excessive inflammation.

Tests for Chronic Inflammation

If your doctor believes inflammation is a problem for you, he or she can order tests that indicate excessive inflammation. Two of the most common are called:

- C-reactive protein (CRP) – this is a blood protein that is considered one of the strongest indicators of inflammation. If your CRP level is high, it indicates inflammation, and possible heart problems, as well as inflammatory disease.
- White blood cell count – white blood cell counts increase in fighting infection. If your white blood cell

count is high and there's no infection present, it can be an indicator of inflammatory disease.

Additional inflammatory marker tests include:

- SED rate – looks for clumping of red blood cells, indicating inflammation.
- Elevated HDL – inflammation impacts HDL levels, quality and effectiveness.
- Elevated blood glucose – the insulin resistance associated with elevated blood glucose also indicates inflammation.
- Homocysteine level – elevated homocysteine level in the blood indicates chemicals that increase inflammation.
- Elevated ferratin in the blood – when inflammation is present, ferratin levels rise.

Dangers of Chronic Inflammation

There's a wide range of effects that chronic inflammation can have for someone suffering from it. This chapter will cover what diseases could be associated with the inflammatory situation in your body. Don't freak out, it's very unlikely you will get most of these diseases.

I highly urge you to consult your local doctor or medical expert, in order to investigate your personal risks on the long term. In itself, inflammation is mostly harmless, but it could be an indicator for something more serious. Always make sure your medical condition is properly researched, if needed with a second opinion from a hospital expert. This book will not be able to indicate for you which diseases you could develop, or might already have developed. For this, a thorough personal medical examination is required.

Inflammation: A Marker for Longevity

How important is it to address chronic inflammation? Consider this: insulin resistance, and the resulting inflammation, are one of the strongest predictors for living a long life. That's right – the presence of chronic inflammation is a clear warning sign that you are at risk for degenerative diseases that will end your life prematurely.

Don't despair. In later chapters, I'll tell you how simple changes in your diet and lifestyle can do a great deal to offset the dangers of inflammation. But first, let's look at the impact chronic inflammation has on your body, and your quality of life.

Associated Autoimmune Disorders

With autoimmune, the body's immune response is in overdrive. With acute, healthy immune responses, the body creates inflammation as part of the healing process, but the inflammation ends once the danger of infection is past. For a variety of reasons, with autoimmune disorders, the inflammation is chronic.

Autoimmune disorders can include:

- Addison's Disease, caused by the adrenal's inability to produce enough hormone;
- Alopecia Areata, in which the immune system attacks hair follicles;
- Antiphospholipid Syndrome, a condition causing problems with the lining of blood vessels, and which can result in blood clots;
- Autoimmune Hepatitis, which attacks and destroys liver cells and can lead to hardening of the liver;
- Celiac Sprue-Dermatitis, a condition in which any gluten eaten results in damage to the small intestine;
- Chronic Fatigue Syndrome Immune Deficiency Syndrome (CFIDS), which results in extreme fatigue;
- Diabetes Type 1, in which the immune system attacks the cells that make insulin, leading to high blood sugar;
- Discoid Lupus, an autoimmune condition that can damage the joints, skin, kidneys, heart, lungs, and more;
- Endometriosis, in which the tissue that generally lines the uterus grows somewhere else in the body;
- Fibromyalgia, a chronic disorder that results in pain, fatigue, and tenderness;
- Grave's Disease, which causes the thyroid to overproduce thyroid hormone;

- Guillain-Barre, which causes the immune system to attach nerves in the brain and spinal cord;
- Hashimoto's Thyroiditis causes the thyroid to under produce hormone;
- Hemolytic Anemia, in which the immune system destroys red blood cells;
- Idiopathic Thrombocytopenia Purpura (ITP), in which the immune system destroys blood platelets needed for clotting;
- Inflammatory Bowel Disease, which causes chronic inflammation of the bowel. IBD includes Crohn's disease, and ulcerative colitis;
- Insulin Dependent Diabetes (Type I), in which the body does not produce enough insulin;
- Juvenile Arthritis, a type of arthritis that affects children 16 and under;
- Meniere's Disease, a disorder of the inner ear;
- Multiple Sclerosis, in which the immune system attacks nerve protective coating, and impacts the brain and spinal cord;
- Myasthenia Gravis, in which the immune system attacks muscles and nerves throughout the body;
- Pemphigus Vulgaris, in which the immune system attacks the skin and forms blisters and sores;
- Pernicious Anemia, caused by an inability to absorb vitamin B-12;

- Polymyositis and Dermatomyositis are inflammatory myopathies that cause muscle inflammation and weakness;
- Primary Agammaglobulinemia; A rare genetic disorder that harms the body's ability to fight infections;
- Primary Biliary Cirrhosis, in which the immune system destroys the liver's bile ducts;
- Psoriasis, in which new skin cells grow too fast and pile up on the surface of the skin;
- Rheumatic Fever, which may develop after a group A Streptococcus bacterial infection;
- Rheumatoid Arthritis, which attacks the lining of the body's joints;
- Scleroderma, in which connective tissue in skin and blood vessels grows abnormally;
- Sjögren's Syndrome, which targets the glands that make moisture, such as the tear ducts;
- Vasculitis, which affects the body's blood vessels;
- Vitiligo, which destroys the cells that provide skin coloration.

Degenerative Diseases Linked to Inflammation

In addition to autoimmune, a number of degenerative diseases have been linked to chronic inflammation, including:

- Alzheimer's disease
- Cancer
- Carpal tunnel
- Depression
- Kidney failure
- Myocardial infarction (heart attack)
- Osteoporosis
- Parkinson's disease
- Stroke
- Tooth decay

Additional Challenges Presented by Inflammation

- You may be slower to heal from injury
- You may be more prone to catch colds and the flu
- You may struggle with allergies and asthma

- You may be more likely to experience complications from surgery, and have slower recovery

Clearly, there are a number of reasons that it's important to address inflammation. Don't be overwhelmed! This book will serve as your guide to reducing chronic inflammation in your life – and feeling great again.

Symptoms of Chronic Inflammation

Identification of the correct symptoms brings you one step closer to a solution. And no – you're not crazy: there is a diagnosis for every weird thing happening in your body. Same thing is true with chronic inflammation.

You can also determine the severity of your inflammation by these symptoms, which is another helpful tool to get your closer to solving your health issues. Moving towards an anti-inflammatory diet is a process: from analysis, to identification, to solving the issues.

A Mantra for Those with Chronic Inflammation

So chronic inflammation is widespread; a growing condition, in Western culture; and a serious threat.

Now the question that matters most: do you have chronic inflammation?

Previously, we mentioned some tests that indicate if inflammation is present in your body. But if you talk to people who have – finally – gotten a diagnosis of chronic inflammation, associated with more specific conditions, most of them will tell you it took a long time, and several physicians, before they got a useful diagnosis. And then, they'll tell you it was difficult to find a medical professional who could give them a path forward on how to live a fulfilling life, with that diagnosis.

There are a number of reasons why people with chronic inflammation and the diseases associated with it can't get an accurate diagnosis, or medication that addresses their condition, or even acknowledgement that their illness is real. "My doctor has been no help and thinks I'm crazy," or statements to that effect, are common. If physicians do diagnose chronic inflammation or an autoimmune disorder, their advice addresses only the *symptoms* – not the disease itself.

If this chapter, and previous chapters, indicate to you that you have chronic inflammation and some form of autoimmune that goes along with chronic inflammation, this should be your mantra:

"My disease is real, and I take responsibility for healing myself."

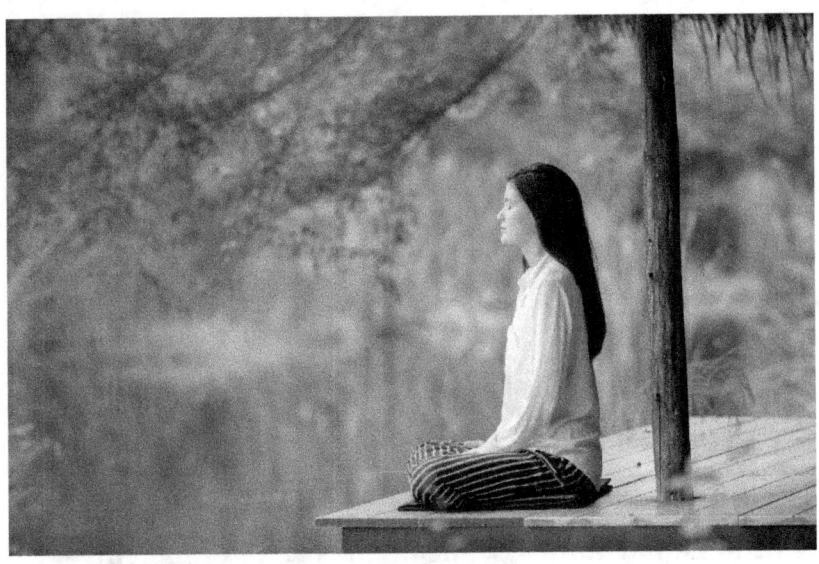

Because the sad truth is – it's very likely you are not going to find a lot of support in the traditional medical community in healing from chronic inflammation and the disorders that accompany it. But here's the good news: in many cases, you *can* go a long way toward healing yourself of chronic inflammation – not with medications or help from the medical community, but with lifestyle changes that you can identify and control, yourself. This book will tell you what you need to know to make those changes – and start feeling better.

Symptoms of Chronic Inflammation

The symptoms of chronic inflammation are often subtle. They worsen over time, and often, slowly – so those who have chronic inflammation may not notice that their quality of life is very gradually worsening. Read over the following list of symptoms to see if the ring true for you. If you suspect you are affected by chronic inflammation, certainly see a medical professional and see if he or she can offer insight, diagnosis and advice. But know also – with many conditions associated with chronic inflammation, you can learn a great deal about your particular condition by making the lifestyle changes in this book, and noticing if you feel different – better.

If, for example, you give up gluten for 21 days and notice your joints ache much less, you have more energy, your skin rashes clear up, and your brain fog clears, you can be relatively certain you have chronic inflammation.

Which of the following symptoms of chronic inflammation are you experiencing?

- Pain in joints or muscles that continues for weeks, with no discernable cause
- Redness and swelling in joints
- Loss of joint function
- Headaches
- Anxiety
- Allergies or asthma that doesn't improve, or is slowly getting worse
- General flu-like symptoms (fever, chills, headache)
- High blood pressure
- High blood sugar

- A reaction to glutinous grains (wheat, barley, or similar)
- Intolerance to heat or cold
- Recurring stomach distress (constipation, diarrhea, bloating, gas, cramps)
- Ongoing fatigue and lethargy
- Difficulty concentrating or focusing
- Skin problems (rashes, white patches, psoriasis, eczema, rosacea)
- Bloodshot eyes
- Dry eyes or mouth
- Insomnia
- Sun sensitivity
- Sores inside mouth
- Hair loss
- Blood or mucous in stool
- Numbness or tingling in extremities
- Multiple miscarriages
- Blood clots

Any of these symptoms could indicate inflammation. If you have them, it's time to move on to shifting your daily diet. Let's look at the diet part of things, shall we?

Diet and Chronic Inflammation

To understand the causes of chronic inflammation and conditions associated with it, it's helpful to keep in mind the definition of chronic inflammation, and the fact that lifestyle choices – particularly diet - impact wellbeing.

There's Still Much to Learn

Chronic inflammation is a condition in which the body attacks itself. Symptoms are almost always improved with changes to lifestyle. That's an indication that chronic inflammation is often brought on by *inflammatory-causing choices in lifestyle* – particularly choices around diet.

And that's a broad range of causes. But it's important to understand the causes of chronic inflammation, in order to remove those causes from your life.

Much of what we know about other diseases is based on medical research and studies. That is not so much true of the wide array of conditions associated with chronic inflammation, for two primary reasons: first, the pharmaceutical industry doesn't usually see much profit in researching and treating chronic inflammation.

In actuality, the drugs for chronic inflammation often have a serious downside, and are not as effective as making changes to your lifestyle. But pharmaceutical companies drive most medical studies, and they don't pursue studies in many of the disorders associated with chronic inflammation.

That means we don't know as much about it as we should; we don't have medications to treat it, often; and (and this is a big one) because Western medicine is more and more driven by pharmaceutical companies, many chronic inflammation/ autoimmune disorders are not recognized as debilitating, either by the government, or even by the medical establishment.

Just ask the 23 million Americans who have chronic inflammation and the disorders associated with it. They'll tell you their struggles in getting treatment and support.

So to understand what causes chronic inflammation and associated disorders: if lifestyle changes are effective in offsetting the symptoms, it follows that, often, lifestyle choices – *primarily diet* - contributed to development of chronic inflammation. Following are factors that experts have identified (or theorized) that cause chronic inflammation and the conditions associated with it:

1. Life in Western cultures has presented the body with more and more infectious agents. As a result, the immune system has been overtaxed, and at some point, may not step away from its role, but continue to attack cells, whether foreign to the body or a part of the body;

2. Increase in environmental toxins and chemicals – many of them in our food - interfere with the way the immune system communicates with the rest of the body. The immune system is no longer

receiving the message that the body is not under attack. The immune system cannot differentiate "self" from "non-self" when it attacks.

Diet and Chronic Inflammation

Studies are increasingly linking diet and choices around diet to the presence of chronic inflammation, from such sources as processed and refined foods, glutens, simple carbohydrates, lectins, saturated fats, omega 6 fatty acids, simple carbohydrates, alcohol and caffeine. Following are specifics about the factors in diet that contribute to chronic inflammation and the diseases associated with chronic inflammation.

Don't assume government regulations are protecting you from food additives in processed foods and fast foods. Pew Research found that eighty percent of the additives in food have not been analyzed regarding their impact on the human body.

Food Additives

A recent study in Israel associates the following food additives with, among other problems, intestinal permeability. When the intestines are more permeable (commonly referred to as "leaky gut"), the leakage is seen by the immune system as attack by foreign bodies. These additives have been shown to significantly affect that response:

Refined salt - Processed foods in the United States have twice as much refined salt as foods in other countries, so the finding that refined salt is one suspected cause of chronic inflammation is particularly significant. A Yale University team found that refined, processed and bleached salts increased the number of cytokines, which in turn affects the myelin, the sheath around nerve fibers, and disrupts messages between brain and body.

Sugars – Sugars contribute to digestive dysfunction and leaky gut syndrome, inflame the endocrine system, and spike insulin.

Emulsifiers – Emulsifiers make it possible to blend substances that generally don't blend – like oil and water – and keep them blended. They are thought to cause pro-inflammatory bacteria from the gut into the body, and produce intestinal inflammation.

Organic Solvents – solvents are used to extract or dissolve substances. They are used in insecticides and in food preparation. In foods, they extract oils from nuts, beans and seeds. Solvents disrupt the communication between brain and body, so the immune system receives false communication to continue attacking, or does not receive communication telling it to stop attacking.

Gluten – Gluten is a protein present in wheat, rye, barley, spelt, and other grains. For many, the immune system perceives gluten as a foreign substance, and becomes inflammatory. *Microbial transglutaminase* is a gluten-derived food protein that thickens and binds processed meat, fish, dairy and baked goods, and that has the same impact on inflammation as other gluten.

Nanometric particles – These are various additives that are thought to improve the uniformity and texture of foods, as well as its taste. Additives such as MSG, food coloring and aspartame are often perceived by the body as foreign substances (which they are), triggering an inflammatory response.

Lectins

Lectins are proteins that bind cellular sugars, keeping them from functioning. Lectins also cause the body to perceive such cells as being foreign, causing an immune system response and inflammation. Lectins are found in saturated fats, certain polyunsaturated fats, alcohol and caffeine, nightshades (tomato, potato and eggplant), gluten, beans and peanuts, dairy and eggs.

Omega 6 Fatty Acids

Omega 6 fatty acids over-stimulate the immune system. They are found in vegetable oils like soy oil, corn oil, and canola. Their impact is worsened when they are heated.

Simple Carbohydrates

Simple carbohydrates are starches and sugars that have a high glycemic impact, meaning they are absorbed into the blood stream quickly. They have been closely linked to development of insulin resistance, and to greater risk of cancer and heart disease. They are sugars (table sugar, corn syrup and honey) and grains (flours that are absorbed quickly into the blood stream).

Trans Fats

Deep fried foods, fast foods and commercially prepared baked goods generally have high levels of trans-fat, as well as hydrogenated oils, margarine and vegetable shortening. Trans-fats promote inflammation, insulin resistance and obesity.

Dairy Products

Yes – this is a painful piece of news for many people. Milk and other dairy are common allergens that can trigger inflammation in the form of cramps, constipation, diarrhea, skin issues, acne, hives and breathing difficulty.

Feedlot-Raised Meat, Red Meat and Processed Meat

Feedlot cattle and other animals are fed soy, corn and bean foods, which are high in Omega-6 fatty acids. Their meat has higher fat levels and contains the antibiotics and hormones they've been given – it gets passed right along to you. All these characteristics are associated with increased inflammation.

Red meat contains the molecule Neu5Gc, which the body responds to with antibodies that may trigger inflammation. Additionally, processed meats contain chemicals, additives and agents linked to cancer.

Alcohol

A high consumption of alcohol often inflames body organs and has been associated with increased risk of cancer.

Your Own Food Intolerances

Your body may respond to particular foods with an inflammatory response. Corn, shellfish, dairy, eggs, tomatoes and peanuts are the foods that most commonly trigger a response, and inflammation. Investigate elimination diets to test what foods may by triggering an inflammatory response in you.

Anti-Inflammatory Diet Success Stories

By now, you may be feeling overwhelmed. It's likely that many of the foods and lifestyle choices we've covered are elements of your everyday life. Well of course they are! They are a primary reason you are experiencing the effects of inflammation!

You're Going to Feel Better

Hang in there. You can do this, and this book is going to be by your side to help. And in the end – you're going to feel better. Physically better, because you've eliminated many of the causes of your inflammation. And psychologically better, because *you* are finally in control of your illness.

You'll find anti-inflammatory diets on the internet and in books that take more risks than this one does. A suggestion: Commit, right now, to giving the next 21 days to finding out *everything* that causes inflammation for *you*. Just 21 days. At the end of it, you'll know exactly what you can feel safe eating – and what foods put you at risk. Let's go over some of the foods that are beneficial to your diet, or that will not cause any inflammation whatsoever. Also, there's a whole list of food you need to test for yourself, and a list of foods you should avoid at all costs.

Anti-Inflammatory Foods: What Will Nourish and Sustain You?

So what can you eat that doesn't trigger inflammation? And what are the foods you cannot eat? I'll break your diet down into:

- Foods that fight inflammation
- Foods that don't lead to inflammation and are allowed
- Foods to test (test to see if they are an issue; if so, eliminate)
- Foods it's best not to eat at all

Foods That Fight Inflammation

These are foods that are your new best friends. Eat these and your inflammation will reduce, or eventually even go away completely. That's true: Not only do they <u>not</u> cause inflammation – they help offset it.

- Fruits (organic strawberries, blueberries, oranges, pineapple and cherries)
- Vegetables (celery, beets, broccoli, leafy greens like kale, spinach, collard greens)
- Nuts (if tolerated) – note that peanuts are not nuts
- Tomatoes, peppers and eggplant (if tolerated)
- Olive oil
- Bone broth
- Wild-caught fatty fish (salmon, mackerel, tuna and sardines)
- Coconut oil
- Turmeric
- Ginger
- Curcuma (see image below)
- Fermented foods (kombucha, sauerkraut, kimchi, fermented vegetables, kefir made with coconut water)
- Avocado

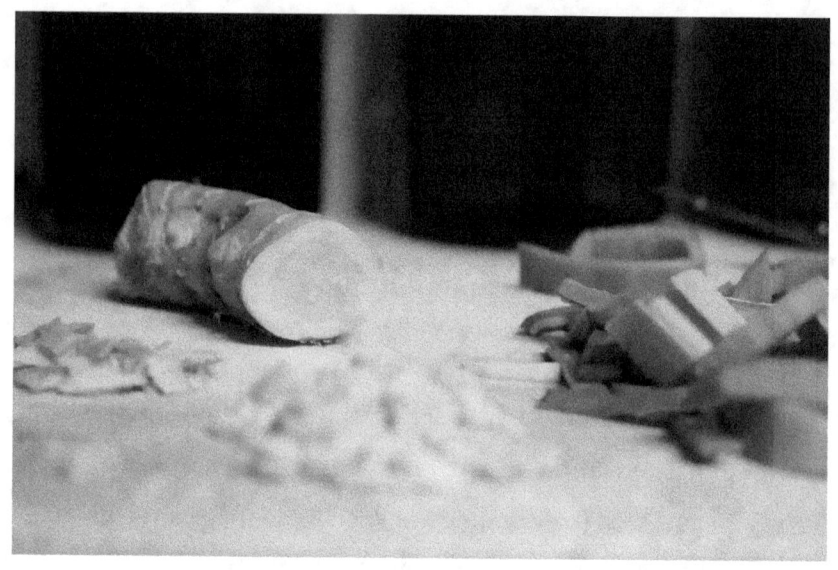

Foods That Don't Trigger Inflammation and Are Allowed

- Allowed vegetables: green beans, peas, leafy vegetables, beets, asparagus, Brussels sprouts, cabbage, broccoli, cauliflower, cucumber, squash, carrots, sweet potatoes
- Fruits
- Wild-caught fish and seafood
- Organic chicken, turkey, boar, game
- Fats – olive oil and coconut oil
- Herbs and spices
- Coconut milk (without additives)

- Non-seed spices (avoid fennel, celery seed, sesame seed, etc.)

Foods to Test

Do not ingest any of these for 21 days. On day 21, choose one thing you eliminated—like dairy or eggs — but not more than one, and eat it. Keep track of how you feel over the next 48 hours. If you have a problem with a food, you'll likely experience one or more of these symptoms: dizziness, stomach cramps, brain fog, fatigue, constipation, diarrhea, headache, bloating, hives.

If you have no reaction after two days, eat that same food again, and again, notice how you feel. If you don't have a reaction, you can make the call on whether to include that food in your diet, or not. Then, pick another food and follow the same steps. Foods to test:

- Non-glutinous whole grains (brown rice, gluten-free oats)
- Legumes (beans)

- Onion
- Grass-fed beef
- Nightshade vegetables (eggplant, tomatoes, peppers)
- Nuts and seeds
- Alcohol (one glass of wine or one mixed drink per day after 21 days, if tolerated. Beer is out of the question, unless it is gluten-free)
- Shellfish
- Eggs

Foods Best Not to Eat At All

- Processed foods
- Processed meats
- Fast food
- Fried food
- Sugars (maple syrup and honey are allowed, once tested)
- Lard
- Butter and margarine
- Canola oil
- Seed oils
- Refined carbohydrates
- Vegetable oils high in Omega-6 (corn, soy, sunflower, safflower, palm)

- Peanuts
- Dairy
- Synthetic sweeteners (Splenda, Aspartame, saccharine)
- Grain-fed meats
- Gluten (wheat, rye and spelt)
- More than one glass of wine or one mixed drink per day
- Trans fat foods (margarine, shortening, commercial baked goods, non-dairy coffee creamers, frozen pizza, microwave popcorn, frosting)
- Additives (watch for guar gum and carrageenan)
- **Any food you are intolerant to** (test to find out)

Don't worry – there are recipes in this book that work for the 21-day elimination period. Again – you can do this. And once you do, it's likely you'll feel so much better that you'll feel glad you did. In fact, many people already did this and have been very successful with their transformation.

And these are ordinary people, just like you and me. So I strongly believe that taking lessons from success stories such as these, helps you succeed as well.

Success Stories

Sam's story

Sam began having pain in his back and knees when he was only seventeen, but back and joint pain ran in his family and he thought it was just an inherited problem that his father had learned to live with – and he would, too. But at 20 he developed psoriasis, and at 22, psoriatic arthritis. He went to three doctors over two months before the psoriatic arthritis was accurately diagnosed.

He began taking recommended medications, but didn't really see a significant improvement until he began eating in accordance with the anti-inflammatory diet. He discovered, through 21 day elimination, that he had a serious food intolerance to nuts and eggs. Eating a diet that eliminated those two foods, as well as inflammation-producing foods, gave him significant improvement in joint pain and psoriasis.

Sam has to be particularly careful during allergy seasons, when his immune system is most taxed, and he's careful not to get stressed and to get enough sleep. He recently went off his medications – a goal he'd had for some time – is on a challenging exercise regimen, and is feeling good.

Rosa's story

Rosa had a slow decline – she first started noticing that she felt cold, even when others complained of the heat. She was fatigued, developed eczema, and frequently caught whatever was going around. She kept asking her physician to help her – he gave her anti-depressants and sent her to a therapist. He felt she was hypochondriac; her mother agreed.

In the next few years, her hair became brittle and much of it fell out. She had no eyebrows. She was swollen, and tired all the time. She had to begin using a cane when she was in her late 30s. She found once she had dressed for the day, she was so tired that for her, the day was essentially over.

Desperate, she committed to the anti-inflammatory diet for 21 days. Within three days, her muscle and joint pain were gone. She saw an integrative doctor who diagnosed her with Hashimoto's; the supplements the physician prescribed, combined with the anti-inflammatory diet, made Rosa actually feel human again.

Thanksgiving that year was hard. Rosa drove the three hours to have Thanksgiving with her family, at her mother's house. She brought much of her own food, to keep her mother from having to make adjustments to the meal. But her mother was offended that Rosa wouldn't eat the food she'd prepared, and implied much of what was challenging Rosa was all in her head. Rosa had a moment of truth when she realized that nothing – nothing – would make her give up the answers she'd found that had changed how terrible she had felt.

The day after Thanksgiving, Rosa told her mother, "It hurts me that you are not supporting me. I don't enjoy having to deny myself your great cooking. But you have to see how much better I am – I'm not using a cane. I'm enrolled in a dance class. I wish you could be happy for me, and support me."

Rosa's mother didn't have much to say, and Rosa drove home determined she'd choose her own health over her mother's needs, if she had to. But the next week, she got a card from her mother in which her mother promised to try to understand, and support her.

It's likely that you, too, will experience challenges – with the medical community, with your food plan, with family or friends. Stick with it. It's your health, and worth whatever other sacrifices you have to meet, or challenges you have to face.

Keys to Making Your Anti-Inflammatory Diet Successful

You are about to embark on a new chapter in your life. In the course of the next few weeks, you'll learn a great deal about yourself – about what's really important to you, and who in your life you can count on to support you.

It's a challenging but exciting adventure. Following in this chapter are some suggestions on how to navigate these changes. And no – you will not always succeed and you WILL divert from your diet at some point. This isn't an issue. The point is, to change your diet over the long term. Eventually, you'll get accustomed to your new food diet.

Just like you get accustomed to another climate when on holiday. It takes some time to adapt, but when you are content in your new situation, you don't want to go back any longer to your old situation.

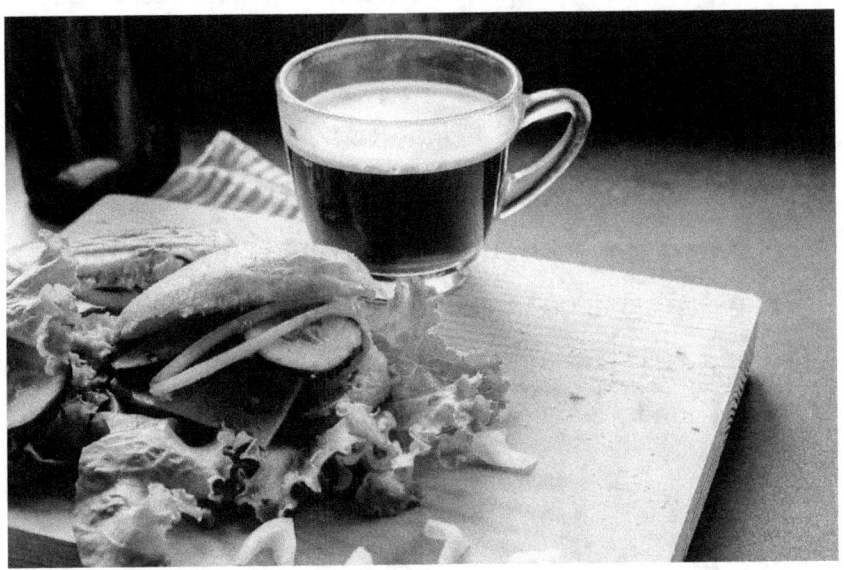

Be With People Who Are Understanding

You are going to need support – people who understand why committing to an anti-inflammatory diet is important to you, and who support you in what you eat – and do their part to cheer you up. Maybe you have friends that are always asking for *your* support. This is an opportunity to see if they'll be there when you need them, too.

If not – well, now you know. Best not to be with those friends or family for the next few weeks. After these changes are second nature to you, you can see those people again – and decide if and to what extent you want to keep them in your life.

Be with people who have a positive attitude, who cheer you up, who support you, but who don't let you play sad sack too much. People who are glad you are doing this – because they want you around, and they want you to feel good again.

Be Flexible

No, not flexible about what you can and cannot eat. But flexible about what a good meal looks like. Breakfast, for example. No eggs? No pancakes? No bacon? Well, what to eat then? Think about it in advance and plan out your healthy meals at the grocery store. That way you will adapt faster.

Though it doesn't sound like breakfast – what about a breakfast hash of chopped baked chicken with chopped sweet potato and apple, with a bit of sage? Your meals may not look like they looked before – but let yourself eat foods you're allowed, that you enjoy, whatever the time of day.

Plan Ahead

Have some food prepared ahead of time to be sure you don't go hungry while you cook – or, worse, to be sure you don't stray from the diet. In particular, cook up some sweet potatoes and have them on hand.

This diet probably has far less carbohydrate than you're used to. Sweet potatoes can help you bridge that change.

Plan what you will cook in the week ahead, and have the ingredients on hand. Give yourself a couple of evenings when you have a simple cold salad – vegetables, oil, lemon juice and some chopped chicken – that's fast, easy and satisfying.

Cover the Basics

In addition to keeping to the food plan, do the following three things. These, and eating anti-inflammatory foods, will likely make a major difference in how you feel – quickly:

- Get plenty of sleep
- Manage your stress with meditation, exercise, avoid what causes stress!
- Exercise
- Be with people you can count on

In a few weeks, you can look at other approaches to bring balance to your life – spirituality, a special interest you can pursue now that you have more energy.

But for now – keeping to the diet, and finding time for these four additional things, is challenge enough. Remember – you can do it, even though it might be difficult at first.

Forego Travel and Social Events If Possible

Travel and social events can challenge your resolve. Avoid them, if you can, for these 21 days. If you must travel or go out, take care of your dietary needs on your own – not with other people – if you can.

Then you can have a simple salad on your own, or just drink a glass of water with lime while everyone else is imbibing alcohol. This is one of the hardest parts, because challenging your old habits in such a situation can be difficult.

Don't Take Dieting Further Than You Need

Now is not the time to restrict your diet further – for example, saying "As long as I'm doing this, I'm going to try to lose 10 pounds as well." Don't set yourself up for failure. The anti-inflammatory diet is challenging, but do-able. Once your 21 days are up, you can turn to additional healthy measures, armed with the knowledge you've gained in watching your reactions to foods.

Commit to Spending What It Takes

Did you know that in 1900 the average American family spent 43% their income on food? Think about that for a minute. We now have so many things we think of as necessities – cell phones, more than one car per family – things have changed. But in 1900, the food supply was also very different. There was much, much less agribusiness spraying food with insecticides and chemicals, poisoning our food for profit. Apples had spots – but they didn't make us sick. Food was grown and sold locally, rather than picked green and sprayed to preserve it and make it ripen at the right time, once it reached the grocery store.

Here it is in a nutshell – it's likely that what we've done to our food is a big part of why you are ill. To get well, you will need to commit to eating like people ate before we began "modernizing" our food growth and processing. That will take more of your time, and cost you more.

You'll likely spend less on eating out. But you'll certainly spend more on groceries. If that's hard to take, here's a suggestion: make a commitment to eating organic (some call it "clean eating") for the next 21 days. See how you feel, and ask yourself if the extra cost is worth it. My prediction is that you'll feel so much better that you'll gladly spend what it takes to nurture yourself, your health and your future.

Recipes and Menus for the Anti-Inflammatory Diet

Now you have all the information about why. This chapter gives you the information about how! It includes three days of meal plans and recipes to get you going on your 21 days of anti-inflammatory diet. Lunches are packable. After you get rolling, you can use the food lists in Chapter 7 (Success Stories) to continue.

Note that, whenever available, the foods you purchase should be organic. If this is not the case, there's a possibility that hormones or other toxic substances could seep into your diet, which is one of the root causes of inflammation. We obviously wish to avoid this.

Your First Three Days: Meal Plan

The table below will give you an overview of a possible diet plan you can follow in a diet that's anti-inflammatory. The dishes included will all help to reduce your symptoms, and possibly reverse any issues you experience with inflammation. Following this 3 day plan will give you a jump into the anti-inflammatory diet. I highly recommend you trying out the meals (some days have multiple options to choose from), and see if you enjoy it.

Furthermore, I highly recommend you to make your own meals using the lists of foods that are good for you (or neutral as far as inflammation issues go), which were provided earlier on in this book.

	Breakfast	**Lunch**	**Dinner**	**Snacks**
Day One	Breakfast salad	Sliced Turkey Rollups Plantain chips	Slow Cooker Herb Chicken Green Beans Cauliflower Cilantro Rice Green Salad	Peaches with cinnamon Small sweet potato with coconut oil, curry powder

Day Two	Spicy Turkey Patties Sliced avocado and grapefruit	Salad greens with diced leftover chicken, olive oil and lemon juice Banana	Citrus Fish Wraps Mashed Sweet Potatoes Steamed broccoli with olive oil and garlic	Apple with lime Plantain Chips Lettuce leaf with chicken and mango
Day Three	Sweet Potato and Sausage Breakfast Hash Cantaloupe with mint	Avocado Tuna Salad Peaches	Chicken Soup with Zucchini Noodles Salad Greens with sliced apple, vegetables of choice, olive oil and apple cider vinegar	Banana with coconut flakes Cucumber with onion and coconut vinegar

Food Prep

You can choose to prep meals ahead, or not; you can set aside a couple of hours and do a lot of prep, or choose to prep the next day's meals after dinner each night of doing this meal plan.

One prep suggestion I have for you that can help alongside most of the meals: bake several sweet potatoes and refrigerate. It's easy to use them in a number of ways quickly if they're pre-cooked.

Prep for Day 1

- Combine all ingredients for breakfast salad except avocado; refrigerate all the foods;
- Make sliced turkey rollups;
- Rice the cauliflower and refrigerate.

Prep for Day 2

- Make spicy turkey patties mixture. You can cook and reheat, or refrigerate mixture until ready to cook;
- Peel and cut up grapefruit;
- Make lunch salad with chicken;
- Prepare vegetables for Citrus Fish Wraps, refrigerate.

Prep for Day 3

- Make Avocado Tuna Salad, omitting the avocado until your meal is ready to eat;
- Prep vegetables for making Chicken Soup.

Recipes

When doing all the meal preps, it's a good idea to already look at the recipes listed below. These are then thing's we will be making and later eating. Let's get rid of that inflammation!

Day 1

Breakfast: **Breakfast Salad** (serves 2)

1 Orange, chopped
1 Banana, sliced
1 stalk celery, chopped
½ C Cucumber, chopped
½ C Jicama or canned water chestnuts, chopped
1 avocado, chopped
1 Tb chopped parsley
Lemon juice
Salt and pepper

Combine ingredients. Simply mix them in a bowl and add spices to your taste. You can make the night before, but wait and add avocado when ready to eat.

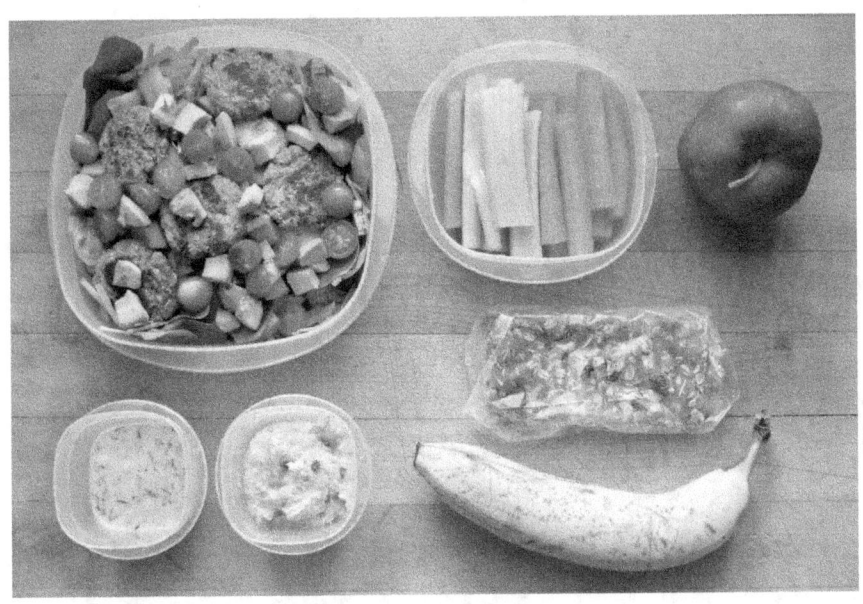

Lunch: **Sliced Turkey Rollups**

2 slices Applegate Farms roasted turkey, sliced thin (get
from deli counter, or use turkey you've roasted)
Shredded cabbage
Shredded carrots
Olive oil with lemon
Sea salt and pepper

Lay turkey slices flat. Fill with ingredients, roll up and
secure with toothpick. Make sure not to use too much
olive oil and salt, as this might be bad to your health.
Be modest with all ingredients.

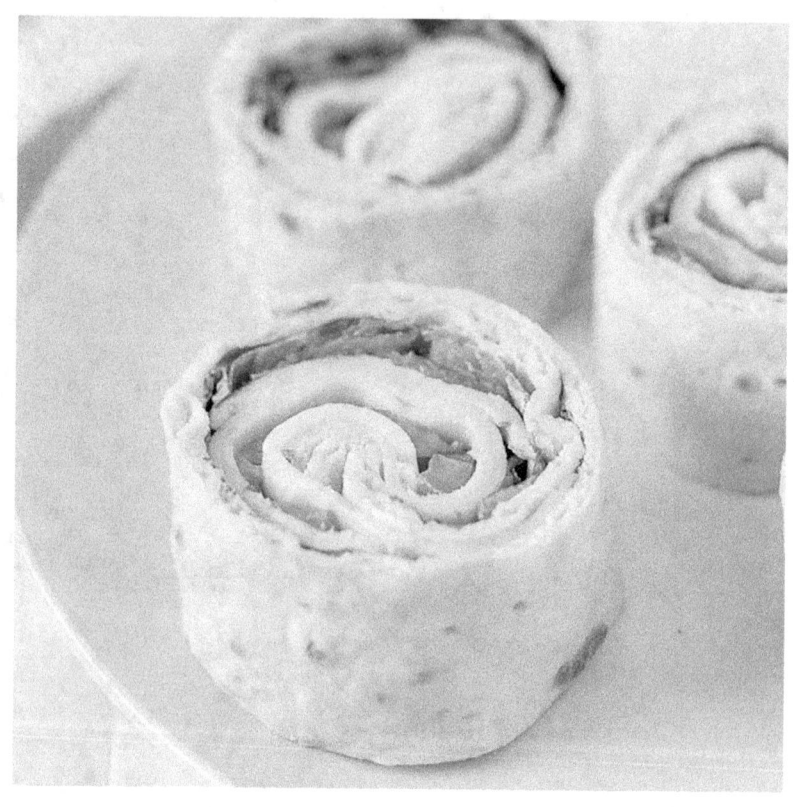

Dinner: **Herbed Slow-Cooker Chicken** (serves 5-6)

2 large white or yellow onions, sliced in rings
6 lbs. organic bone-in chicken thighs, skin removed
4 TB Olive Oil
20 garlic cloves
4 tsp sea salt
2 tsp Italian herbs (just the herbs! No additives!)
2 tsp ground pepper

1. Place the sliced onions in the bottom of a 6-quart slow cooker. (If you are making half this recipe, and your slow cooker is larger, put ingredients in a smaller, oven-proof dish that will fit inside the slow cooker.)

2. Smash the garlic cloves with the side of a knife, peel, and place in a mixing bowl. Add the olive oil and chicken; stir to coat the chicken. Add the sea salt, herbs and pepper, and stir to coat the chicken.

3. Transfer the chicken mixture to the slow cooker, placing it on top of the onions.

4. Cook on low for 6 hours or on high for 4 hours (adjust time for the characteristics of your slow cooker)

5. Reserve leftover chicken to use on Day 2 lunch and Day 3 dinner. Note: when cooking chicken in the slow cooker, thighs do better than chicken breasts (and cost less too!). Sauce in image is optional.

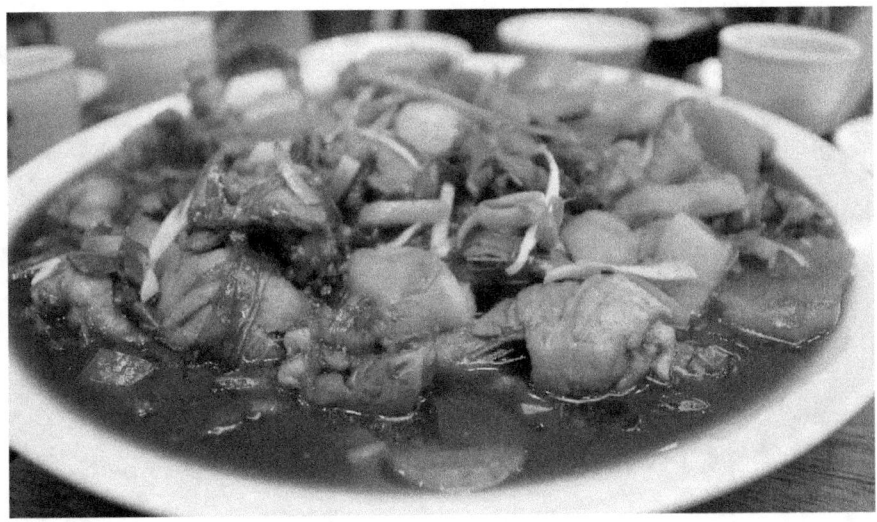

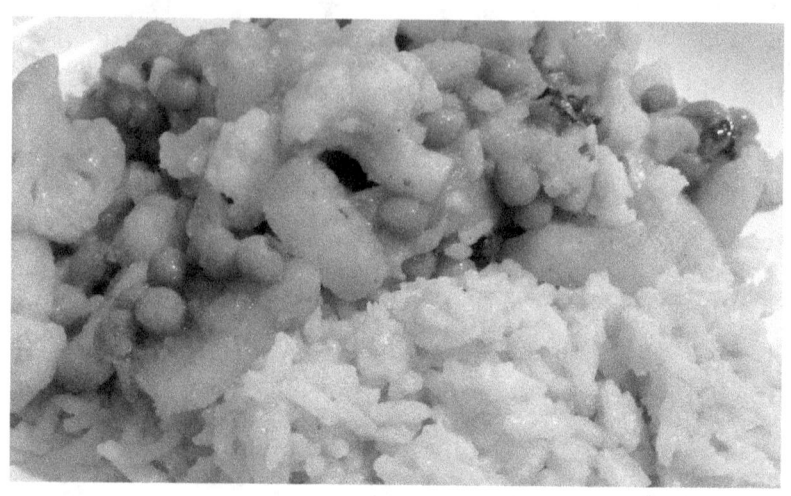

Dinner: **Cauliflower Cilantro Rice** (serves 4)

1 head cauliflower, cut into florets
2 Tb olive oil
½ C diced onion
¾ tsp sea salt
½ tsp dried parsley, garlic powder
¼ tsp ground pepper
¼ tsp cumin
1/3 C organic chicken broth
¼ C minced cilantro

1. Put half the cauliflower florets in food processor and pulse until grainy, like rice. Set aside and pulse other half of the florets.

2. Heat olive oil in a sauté pan. Add onion and cook until onion is translucent. Add salt, parsley, garlic powder, pepper and cumin and cook 1 minute.

3. Add cauliflower and sauté for 5 minutes.
4. Add chicken broth & cilantro. Cover the skillet, steam for 5 minutes.

Day 2

This day is a great moment to reuse some leftovers from the previous meals. So that's what we are going to do. Let's start with some delicious turkey...

Breakfast: **Spicy Turkey Sausage**

2 lbs organic ground turkey or chicken
2 cloves garlic, minced
2 Tb. dried sage
1.5 tsp dried thyme
Pinch nutmeg
1 Tb sea salt
1 tsp ground pepper
4 tsp olive oil

Mix together all ingredients except oil. Refrigerate for at least 15 minutes. Shape into patties and fry. Use leftovers in Day 3's Breakfast Hash.

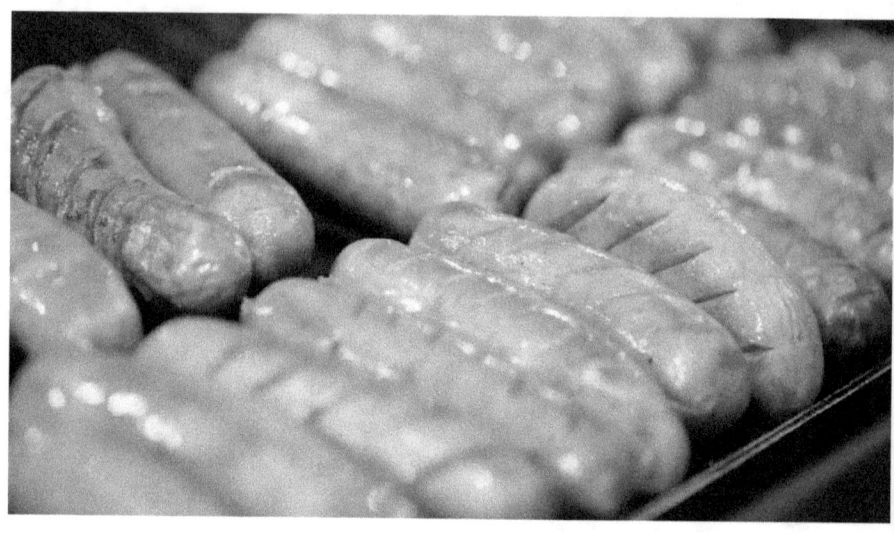

Dinner: **Citrus Fish Wraps** (serves 4)

1 Tb olive oil
2 cups chopped kale, chard or spinach
1 cup carrots, cut into strips
1 celery stalk, sliced
4 Tb chopped scallions (divided)
1 tsp dried Italian herbs
Juice and zest of 1 large orange (finely grate *only* the orange part of the peel).
Salt and pepper to taste
1 Lb frozen wild-caught white fish fillets, thawed

1.   Preheat your oven to 450°F;

2. Heat oil in a large sauté pan and cook kale, carrots, celery and 2 Tb of the scallions until soft, about 7 minutes;

3. Let cool, and toss with herbs, orange juice and orange zest;

4. Line a baking dish with enough foil to fold and crimp closed;

5. Spoon 2 Tb of the orange/vegetable filling onto each fillet. Gently roll up, secure with toothpicks;

6. Arrange the ingredients in a pan; top with remaining orange/vegetable mixture;

7. Fold foil & crimp edges closed. Bake 14 minutes. Sprinkle with remaining scallions.

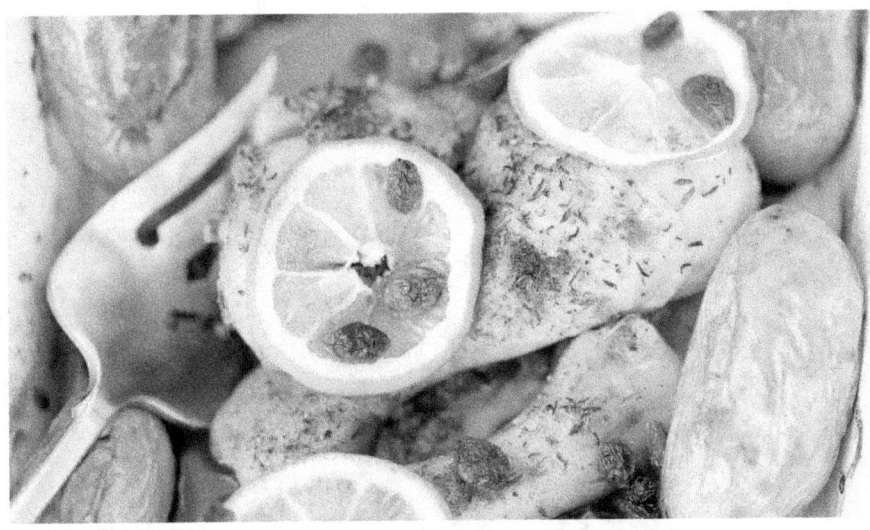

Day 3

Breakfast: **Sweet Potato Breakfast Hash** (serves 2)

1 shallot, thinly sliced
1 unpeeled apple, chopped
2 stalks kale or chard, center ribs removed, cut into ribbons
2 C pre-cooked sweet potato, chopped
4 Leftover Spicy Turkey Sausage patties, chopped
Dried thyme
1 Tb olive oil

Heat olive oil in a skillet. Add shallot, apple and kale and sauté for 2 minutes. Add sweet potato, turkey and thyme. Heat for 2 minutes and serve. You can easily double this recipe to serve 4. You can also replace turkey with prawn like image shown below.

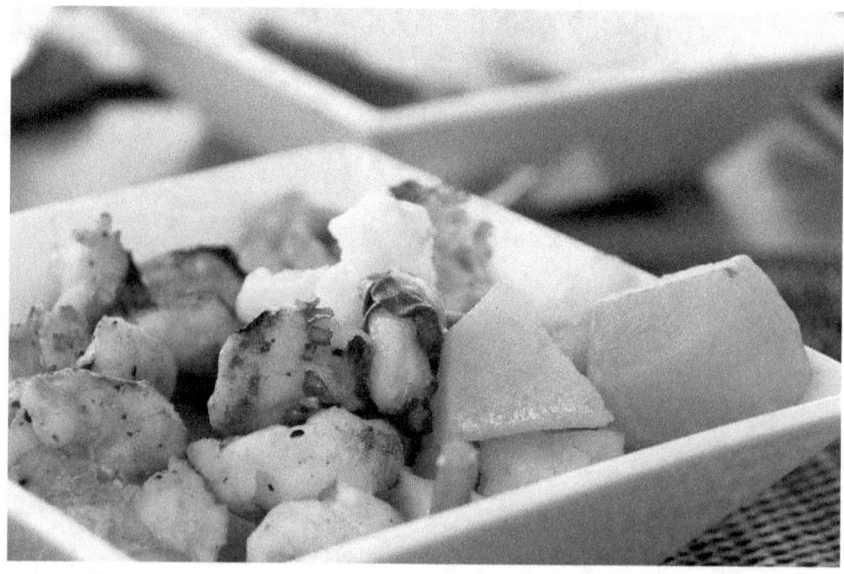

Lunch: **Avocado Tuna Salad** (serves 4)

2 Cans solid white Albacore tuna in water, drained
2 avocados, diced
½ C diced cucumber
2 Tb chopped green onion
1/3 C chopped cilantro
1 Orange, diced
½ tsp garlic salt
Juice from ½ lime
Sea salt and pepper

Simply combine the ingredients in a bowl, mix them
and refrigerate them before use.

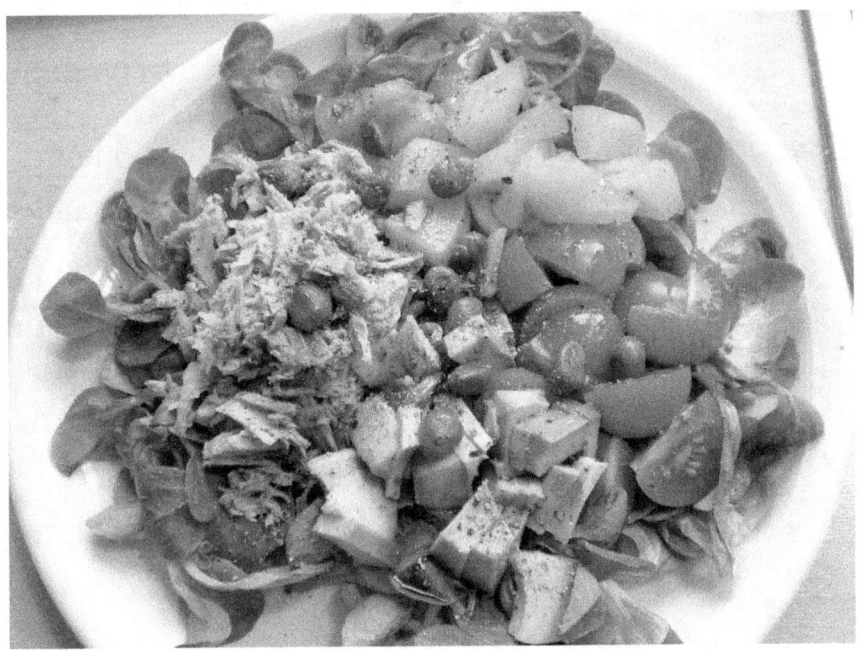

Dinner: **Chicken Soup with Zucchini Noodles** (serves 4)

7 cups Organic Chicken Broth (home-made, or purchased)
2 cups shredded organic chicken (from Day 1 Slow Cooker Chicken)
2 Tb. Olive Oil
2 stalks organic celery, diced
2 organic carrots, diced
3 oz. sliced mushrooms
1 white or yellow onion, chopped
1 shallot, chopped
2 bay leaves
½ tsp dried thyme
2 Tb fresh parsley, chopped (or 1 Tb dried)
Sea salt and ground pepper to taste
2 Zucchini, peeled and cut into thin ribbons (or use a spiralizer to cut into noodles)

1. Place olive oil in a stock pot and heat for a minute or so. Add celery, carrots, mushrooms, onion and shallot. Sauté on low heat until vegetables soften and onion is translucent.

2. Add the broth, bay leaves and thyme. Bring to a boil, then lower heat and cook for 10 minutes.

3. Add shredded chicken and zucchini noodles. Bring to a gentle boil and cook for 5 minutes on low heat. Remove bay leaves, add parsley, season with salt and pepper.

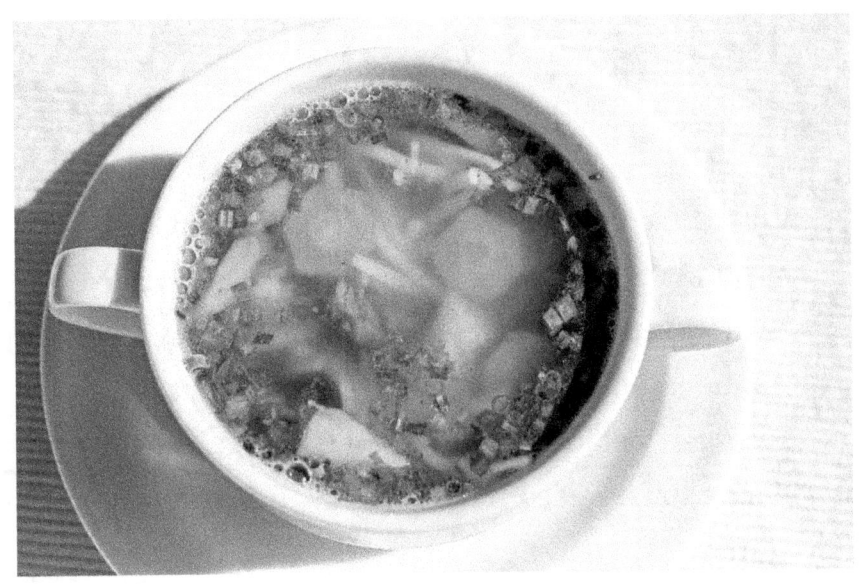

These are just some of the possible meals you can eat when you are trying to go anti-inflammatory.

However, combinations are endless and with the types of foods indicted in this book, you can create your own amazing dishes in no-time. We provided you with the first few days, now it's up to you to go ahead and get create with some of the other foods out there that are good for you!

Parting Words

With these final words, this short guidebook on the anti-inflammatory diet comes to a conclusion. We have looked at the entire process, from root causes to solutions, and everything in between. I have thoroughly enjoyed creating this short guidebook, and I hope you have learned something from it!

Changing your lifestyle in any way is often a difficult and time-consuming thing. However, the results can be very rewarding, even when it comes to the little things. By now, you know what foods to avoid and which ones to embrace: a long process of change awaits you with this newly found knowledge.

Making a start is 50% of the work, I truly believe that. Once you make the shift in your mindset, actively wanting to change your life for the better, is a profound decision that will help you on your path to a healthier life. The inspiration of the success stories will motivate you to success, I hope.

For now, I wish to sincerely thank you for your time spent reading this book. It was a great pleasure to create, and hopefully also a great pleasure to read. Best of luck to you and make sure to keep an eye out for some of the diet-related books I'm about to publish in the near future.

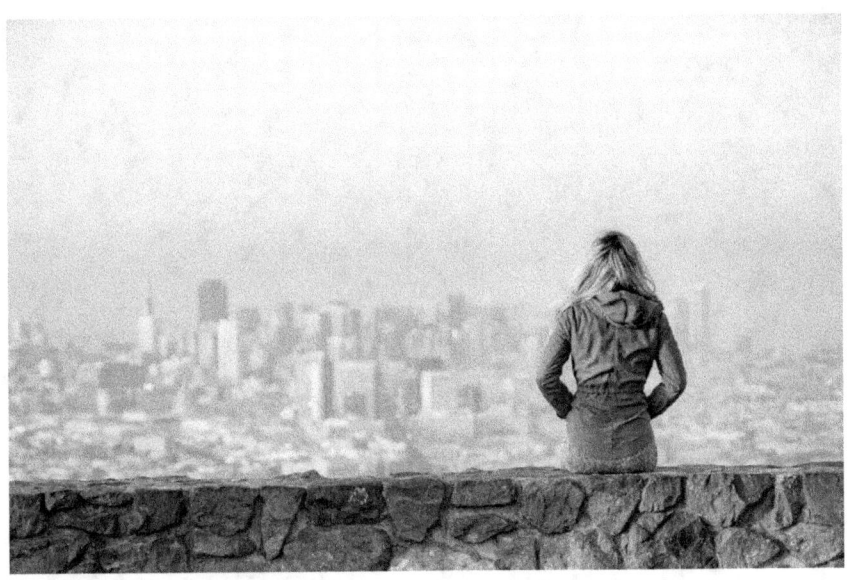

Stephany J. Greene

Author

www.ingramcontent.com/pod-product-compliance
Lightning Source LLC
Chambersburg PA
CBHW062059280526
45788CB00003B/1285